Sirtfood Diet Snack and Dessert

Best Sirtfood Snack and Dessert Recipes

Sommario

Introduction

Thinking about the concept of diet in recent times are based on fasting, this diet instead is not based on a drastic reduction of calories but at the same time you should not give up the results. his type of diet is based on the intake of certain foods that allow you to lose weight faster allowing you to lose weight up to 3 kg per week.A false belief of modern diets is the impossibility of eating snak or sweets but thanks to this diet you will see that it is absolutely not so, enjoy delighting in these recipes for you and your family without giving up weight loss and better physical strength.If you are hesitant about this fantastic diet you just have to try it and analyze your results in a short time, trust me you will be satisfied.Always remember that the best way to lose weight is to analyze your situation with the help of a professional.

Chapter 1 Snacks

Lemongrass Green Tea

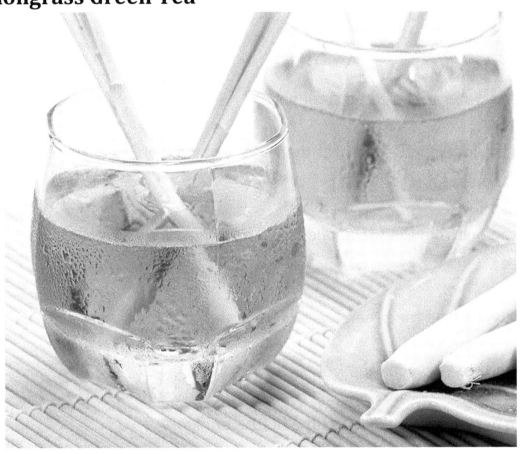

Preparation time: 3 minutes
Cooking time: 12 min
Servings: 1

Ingredients:

Two teaspoons cleaved lemongrass

One teaspoon green tea leaves

1 cup of water

One teaspoon nectar

Directions:

Move the water to a treated steel pot.

Hurl in the lemongrass and heat the water to the point of boiling. Let it bubble for 5 minutes.

Expel the pot from the fire and let the water cool till the temperature is 80-85 degrees C.

Presently, include the green tea and let it soak for 3 minutes.

Strain the tea into your cup.

Include nectar and mix a long time before drinking.

Nutrition:

Calories: 2.5 Calcium: 3mg

Potassium: 34mg Magnesium: 2.9g

Grape and Melon Juice

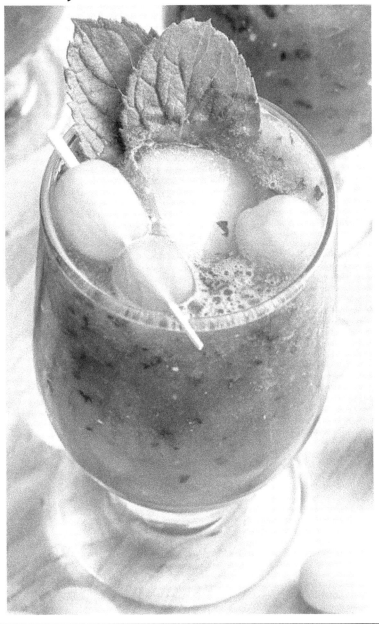

Preparation time: 10 minutes
Cooking time: 0 minutes
Servings: 1

Ingredients:

½ cucumber, stripped whenever liked, split, seeds evacuated and generally slashed

30g youthful spinach leaves stalks expelled

100g red seedless grapes

100g melon, stripped, deseeded

Directions:

Cut into pieces. Blend in a juicer or blender until smooth.

Nutrition:

Calories: 125

Net carbs: 31.7g

Fat: 0.24g

Protein: 0.63g

Kale and Blackcurrant Smoothie

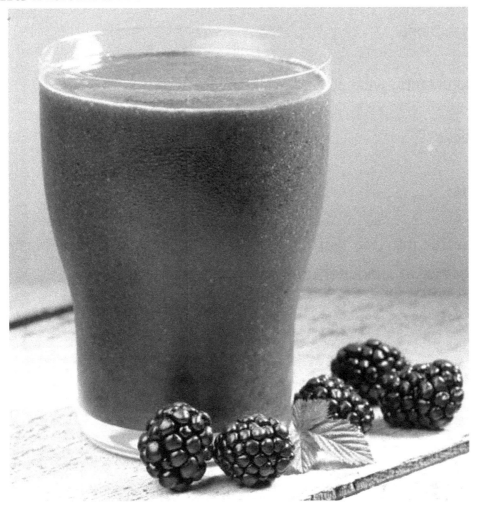

Preparation time: 10 minutes
Cooking time: 0 minutes
Servings: 2

Ingredients:

2 teaspoon nectar

1 cup crisply made green tea

Ten infant kale leaves stalk expelled

One ready banana

40 g blackcurrants, washed and stalks evacuated

Six ice blocks

Directions:

Mix the nectar into the warm green tea until disintegrated. Master all the fixings together in a blender until smooth. Serve right away.

Nutrition:

Calories: 86

Net carbs: 32.9g

Protein: 4.5g

Kale, Edamame and Tofu Curry

Preparation time: 5 minutes
Cooking time: 8 minutes
Servings: 4

Ingredients:

1 teaspoon rapeseed oil

One huge onion, cleaved

Four cloves garlic stripped and ground

One massive thumb (7cm) crisp ginger, stripped and ground

One red bean stew, deseeded and meagerly cut

1/2 teaspoon ground turmeric

1/4 teaspoon cayenne pepper

1 teaspoon paprika 1 teaspoon salt

1/2 teaspoon ground cumin

250g dried red lentils 1-litre bubbling water

50g solidified soy edamame beans

200g firm tofu, cleaved into solid shapes

Two tomatoes, generally cleaved

Juice of 1 lime

200g kale leaves stalks expelled and torn

Directions:

Put the oil in an overwhelming bottomed container over a low-medium warmth. Include the onion and cook for 5 minutes before including the garlic, ginger and stew and preparing for a further 2 minutes. Include the turmeric, cayenne, paprika, cumin and salt. Mix through before including the red lentils and blending once more.

pour in the bubbling water and bring to a generous stew for 10 minutes, at that point decrease the warmth and cook for a further 20-30 minutes until the curry has a thick '•porridge' consistency.

Add the soya beans, tofu and tomatoes and cook for a further 5 minutes. Include the lime juice and kale leaves and cook until the kale merely is delicate.

Nutrition: Protein: 12.6g

Calories: 342 Net carbs: 8.4g Fat: 17g

Green Tea Smoothie

Preparation time: 10 minutes
Cooking time: 0 minutes
Servings: 2

Ingredients:

Two ready bananas 250 ml of milk

2 teaspoon matcha green tea powder

1/2 teaspoon vanilla bean glue (not separate) or a little scratch of the seeds from a vanilla unit

Six ice blocks 2 teaspoon nectar

Directions:

Just mix all the fixings in a blender and serve in two glasses.

Nutrition:

Calories: 183 Net carbs: 33g Fat: 0.6g

Fiber: 3.8g Protein: 2.1g

Sirt Muesli

Preparation time: 10 minutes
Cooking time: 0 minutes
Servings: 2

Ingredients:

20g buckwheat flakes sirtfood plans

10g buckwheat puffs

15g parched coconut

40g Medjool dates, hollowed and cleaved

15g pecans, cleaved

10g cocoa nibs

100g strawberries, hulled and cleaved

100g plain Greek yoghurt (or veggie lover elective, for example, soya or coconut yoghurt)

Directions:

Blend the entirety of the above fixings, possibly including the yoghurt and strawberries before serving on the off chance that you are making it in mass.

Nutrition:

Calories: 25

Net carbs: 43.3g

Fat: 7.2g

Fiber: 6.5g

Protein: 9.0g

Fruit Salad

Preparation time: 10 min
Cooking time: 0 minutes
Servings: 1

Ingredients:

½ cup crisply made green tea

1 teaspoon nectar One orange, split

One apple, cored and generally cleaved

Ten red seedless grapes

Ten blueberries

Directions:

Stir the nectar into a large portion of some green tea. At the point when broken up, include the juice of a large part of the orange. Leave to cool.

Chop the other portion of the orange and spot in a bowl together with the hacked apple, grapes and blueberries. Pour over the cooled tea and leave to soak for a couple of moments before serving.

Nutrition: Calories: 157 Net carbs: 13g

Fiber: 1g Protein: 0.5g

Golden Turmeric Latte

Preparation time: 3 minutes
Cooking time: 7 minutes
Servings: 3

Ingredients:

3 cups of coconut milk

One teaspoon turmeric powder

One teaspoon cinnamon powder

One teaspoon crude nectar

Directions:

Spot of dark pepper (expands retention)

Modest bit of new stripped ginger root

Place of cayenne pepper (discretionary)

Mix all fixings in a fast blender until smooth.

Fill a little container and warmth for 4 minutes over medium heat until hot however not bubbling.

Nutrition:

Calories: 50

Net carbs: 98g

Fat: 2.7g

The Sirt Juice

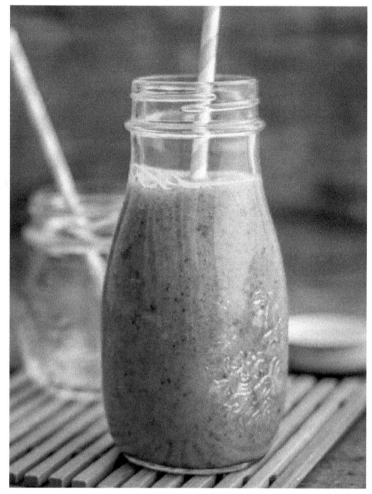

Preparation time: 7-8 min
Cooking time: 0 minutes
Servings: 2

Ingredients:

Two huge bunches (75g) kale

A huge bunch (30g) rocket

A tiny bunch (5g) level leaf parsley

A small bunch (5g) lovage leaves (discretionary)

2–3 huge stalks (150g) green celery, including its leaves

½ medium green apple

Juice of ½ lemon

½ level teaspoon matcha green tea

Directions:

Blend the greens (kale, rocket, parsley and lovage, on the off chance that was utilizing), at that point juice them. We discover juicers can indeed vary in their effectiveness at squeezing verdant vegetables, and you may need to re-squeeze the leftovers before proceeding onward to different fixings. The objective is to wind up with about 50ml of juice from the greens.

Presently squeeze the celery and apple. You can strip the lemon and put it through the juicer also, however, we think that it's a lot simpler just to crush the lemon by hand into the juice. By this stage, you ought to have around 250ml of milk altogether, maybe marginally more. It is just when the sauce is made and prepared to serve that you include the matcha green tea.

Pour a limited quantity of the juice into a glass, at that point include the matcha and mix enthusiastically with a fork or teaspoon. We just use matcha in the first two beverages of the day as it contains reasonable measures of caffeine (a similar substance as a typical cup of tea). For individuals not accustomed to it, it might keep them wakeful whenever alcoholic late once the match is broken up, including the rest of the juice.

Give it a last mix; at that point, your juice is prepared to drink. Don't hesitate to top up with plain water, as indicated by taste.

Nutrition:

Calories: 75

Net carbs: 3.8g

Fat: 0.6g

Fiber: 2.9g

Protein: 0.4g

Kale Pesto Hummus

Preparation time: 10 minutes
Cooking time: 7 minutes
Servings: 12

Ingredients:

Chickpeas, drained and liquid reserved – 15 ounces

Reserved chickpea liquid - .25 cup

Sea salt - .5 teaspoon

Tahini paste - .5 cup

Garlic, minced – 2 cloves

Lemon juice – 2.5 s

Extra virgin olive oil - .33 cup

Black pepper, ground - .5 teaspoon

Kale, chopped and leaves packed – 2 cups

Pine nuts – 2 s

Basil leaves, packed – 1.25 cups

Garlic, minced – 4 cloves

Extra virgin olive oil - .25 cup

Directions:

Into a food processor add the basil, kale, pine nuts, and four cloves of minced garlic. Pulse until the leaves and garlic are finely chopped.

Pour in the olive oil, and once again pulse until smooth. Remove the pesto from the bowl of the food processor and set aside.

Into the empty food processor add the remaining ingredients to assemble the hummus, pulsing until creamy. Add in the prepared pesto, and pulse just until the two are combined.

Transfer the pesto hummus to a serving bowl or store in the fridge.

Nutrition:

Calories: 194 Net carbs: 3.8g

Fat: 2.2g Fiber: 1.8g Protein: 5.6g

Parsley Hummus

Preparation time: 5 minutes
Cooking time: 7 minutes
Servings: 6

Ingredients:

Chickpeas, drained and rinsed – 15 ounces

Curly parsley, stems removed – 1 cup

Sea salt – .5 teaspoon

Soy milk, unsweetened - .5 cup

Extra virgin olive oil – 3 teaspoons

Lime juice – 1 s

Red pepper flakes -.5 teaspoons

Black pepper, ground - .25 teaspoon

Pine nuts – 2 s

Sesame seeds, toasted – 2 s

Directions:

In the food processor pulse the parsley and toasted sesame seeds until it forms a fine powdery texture. Drizzle in the extra virgin olive oil in while you continue to pulse, until it is smooth.

Add the chickpeas, lime juice, and seasonings to the food processor and pulse while slowly adding in the soy milk. Continue to pulse the parsley hummus until it is smooth and creamy.

Adjust the seasonings to your preference and then serve or refrigerate the hummus.

Nutrition: Calories: 107 Net carbs: 7.7g

Fat: 4.5g Fiber: 0.2g Protein: 8.6g

Edamame Hummus

Preparation time: 7 minutes
Cooking time: 0 minutes
Servings: 10

Ingredients:

Edamame, cooked and shelled – 2 cups

Sea salt – 1 teaspoon

Extra virgin olive oil – 1

Tahini paste - .25 cup

Lemon juice - .25 cup

Garlic, minced – 3 cloves

Black pepper, ground - .25 teaspoon

Directions:

Add the cooked edamame and remaining ingredients to a blender or food processor and mix on high until it forms a creamy and completely smooth mixture. Taste it and adjust the seasonings to your preference.

Serve the hummus immediately with your favorite vegetables or store in the fridge.

Nutrition:

Calories: 88

Net carbs: 3.8g

Protein: 2.6g

Edamame Guacamole

Preparation time: 7 minutes
Cooking time: 0 minutes
Servings: 6

Ingredients:

Edamame, cooked and shelled – 1 cup

Avocado, pitted and halved – 1

Red onion, diced - .5 cup

Cilantro, chopped - .25 cup

Jalapeno, minced – 1

Garlic, minced – 2 cloves

Lime juice – 2 s Water – 3 s

Lime zest - .5 teaspoon

Roma tomato, diced – 2

Cumin - .125 teaspoon

Sea salt - .5 teaspoon

Directions:

Into a blender or food processor add all of the ingredients, except for the diced tomato, onion, and jalapeno. Blend the tomato mixture on high speed until it is smooth and creamy, making sure that the edamame has been completely blended.

Adjust the seasoning to your preference and then transfer the guacamole to a serving bowl. Stir in the tomato, onion, and jalapeno. Place the bowl in the fridge, allowing it to chill for at least thirty minutes before serving.

Nutrition: Calories: 100 Net carbs: 13g

Fat: 6.6g Fiber: 6.2g Protein: 45g

Eggplant Fries with Fresh Aioli

Preparation time: 10 minutes
Cooking time: 25 minutes
Servings: 4

Ingredients:

Eggplants – 2

Black pepper, ground - .25 teaspoon

Extra virgin olive oil – 2 s

Cornstarch – 1

Basil, dried – 1 teaspoon

Garlic powder - .25 teaspoon

Sea salt - .5 teaspoon

Mayonnaise, made with olive oil - .5 cup

Garlic, minced – 1 teaspoon

Basil, fresh, chopped – 1

Lemon juice – 1 teaspoon

Chipotle, ground - .5 teaspoon

Sea salt - .25 teaspoon

Directions:

Begin by preheating your oven to Fahrenheit four-hundred and twenty-five degrees. Place a wire cooking/cooling rack on a baking sheet.

Remove the peel from the eggplants and then slice them into rounds, each about three-quarters of an inch thick. Slice the rounds into wedges one inch in width.

Add the eggplant wedges to a large bowl and toss them with the olive oil. Once coated, add the pepper, cornstarch, dried basil, garlic powder, and sea salt, tossing until evenly coated.

Arrange the eggplant wedges on top of the wire rack and set the baking sheet in the oven, allowing the fries to cook for fifteen to twenty minutes.

Meanwhile, prepare the aioli. To do this, add the remaining ingredients into a small bowl and whisk them together to combine. Cover the bowl of aioli and allow it to chill it in the fridge until the fries are ready to be served.

Remove the fries from the oven immediately upon baking, or allow them to cook under the broiler for an additional three to four minutes for extra crispy fries. Serve immediately with the aioli.

Nutrition:

Calories: 243

Net carbs: 12.6g

Fat: 0.5g

Fiber: 13.2g

Protein: 5.3g

Eggplant Caponata

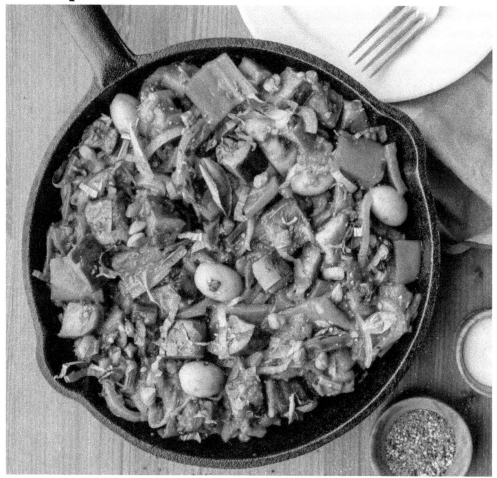

Preparation time: 10 minutes
Cooking time: 25 minutes
Servings: 4

Ingredients:

Eggplant, sliced into 1.5-inch cubes – 1 pound

Bell pepper, diced – 1

Green and black olives, chopped - .5 cup

Capers - .25 cup

Sea salt – 1 teaspoon

Garlic, minced – 4

Red onion, diced – 1

Diced tomatoes – 15 ounces

Extra virgin olive oil – 4 s, divided

Black pepper, ground - .25 teaspoon

Parsley, chopped - .25 cup

Directions:

Preheat your oven to Fahrenheit four-hundred degrees and line a baking sheet with kitchen parchment.

Toss the eggplant cubes in half of the olive oil and then arrange them on the baking sheet, sprinkling the sea salt over the top. Allow the eggplant to roast until tender, about twenty minutes.

Meanwhile, add the remaining olive oil into a large skillet along with the red onions, bell pepper, diced tomatoes, and garlic. Sautee the vegetables until tender, about ten minutes.

Add the roasted eggplant, capers, olives, and black pepper to the skillet, continuing to cook together for five minutes so that the flavors meld.

Remove the skillet from the heat, top it off with parsley, and serve it with crusty toast.

Nutrition:

Calories: 209 Net carbs: 1.6g Fat: 2.3g

Fiber: 5.4g Protein: 0.3g

Buckwheat Crackers

Preparation time: 10 minutes
Cooking time: 1 hour
Servings: 12

Ingredients:

Buckwheat groats – 2 cups

Flaxseeds, ground - .75 cup

Sesame seeds - .33 cup

Sweet potatoes, medium, grated – 2

Extra virgin olive oil – .33 cup

Water – 1 cup

Sea salt – 1 teaspoon

Directions:

Soak the buckwheat groats in water for at least four hours before preparing the crackers. Once done soaking, drain off the water.

Preheat the oven to a temperature of Fahrenheit three-hundred and fifty degrees, prepare a baking sheet, and set aside some kitchen parchment and plastic wrap.

In a kitchen bowl, combine the ground flaxseeds with the warm water, allowing the seeds to absorb the water and form a substance similar to gelatin. Add the buckwheat groats and other remaining ingredients.

Spread the cracker dough onto a sheet of kitchen parchment and cover it with a sheet of plastic wrap. Use a rolling pen on top of the plastic wrap (so that it doesn't stick) and roll out the buckwheat cracker dough until it is thin.

Peel the plastic wrap off of the crackers and transfer the dough-coasted sheet of kitchen parchment to the prepared baking sheet. Allow it to partially bake for fifteen minutes and then remove the tray from the oven.

Reduce the oven temperature to Fahrenheit three-hundred degrees. Use a pizza cutter and slice the crackers into squares, approximately two inches in width. Return the crackers to the oven until they are crispy and dry, about thirty-five to forty minutes.

Remove the crackers from the oven, allowing them to cool completely before storing them in an air-tight container.

Nutrition:

Calories: 158

Net carbs: 6.6g

Fat: 3.8g

Fiber: 2.6g

Protein: 3.4g

Matcha Protein Bites

Preparation time: 15 minutes
Cooking time: 70 minutes
Servings: 12

Ingredients:

Almond butter - .25 cup

Matcha powder – 2 teaspoons

Soy protein isolate – 1 ounce

Rolled oats - .5 cup

Chia seeds – 1

Coconut oil – 2 teaspoons

Honey – 1

Sea salt - .125 teaspoon

Directions:

In a food processor combine all of the matcha protein bite ingredients until it forms a mixture similar to wet sand, that will stick together when squished between your fingers.

Divide the mixture into twelve equal portions. You can do this by eye while estimating, or you can use a digital kitchen scale if you want the portions to be exact. Roll each portion between the palms of your hands to form balls.

Chill the bites in the fridge for up to two weeks.

Nutrition:

Calories: 164 Net carbs: 13.3g

Fat: 4.7g Fiber: 1.2g Protein: 4.5g

Chocolate-Covered Strawberry Trail Mix

Preparation time: 5 minutes
Cooking time: 0 minutes
Servings: 10

Ingredients:

Freeze-dried strawberries – 1 cup

Dark chocolate chunks - .66 cup

Walnuts, roasted – 1 cup

Almonds, roasted - .25 cup

Cashews, roasted - .25 cup

Directions:

Mix together all of the trail mix ingredients in a bowl, and then store it in a large glass jar or divide each serving into its own transportable plastic bag. Store for up to one month.

Nutrition:

Calories: 164

Net carbs: 17.2g

Fat: 3.2g

Fiber: 6.7g

Protein: 2.2g

Moroccan Spiced Eggs

Preparation time: 1 hour 10 minutes
Cooking time: 45 minutes
Servings: 2

Ingredients:

1 tablespoon olive oil

One shallot, stripped and finely hacked

One red (chime) pepper, deseeded and finely hacked

One garlic clove, stripped and finely hacked

One courgette (zucchini), stripped and finely hacked

1 tablespoon tomato puree (glue)

½ teaspoon gentle stew powder

¼ teaspoon ground cinnamon

¼ teaspoon ground cumin

½ teaspoon salt

400g can hacked tomatoes

400g may chickpeas in water

A little bunch of level leaf parsley cleaved

Four medium eggs at room temperature

Directions:

Heat the oil in a pan, include the shallot and red (ringer) pepper and fry delicately for 5 minutes. At that point include the garlic and courgette (zucchini) and cook for one more moment or two. Include the tomato puree (glue), flavors and salt and mix through.

Add the cleaved tomatoes and chickpeas (dousing alcohol and all) and increment the warmth to medium. With the top of the dish, stew the sauce for 30 minutes – ensure it is delicately rising all through and permit it to lessen in volume by around 33%.

Remove from the warmth and mix in the cleaved parsley.

Preheat the grill to 200C/180C fan/350F.

When you are prepared to cook the eggs, bring the tomato sauce up to a delicate stew and move to a little broiler confirmation dish.

Crack the eggs on the dish and lower them delicately into the stew. Spread with thwart and prepare in the grill for 10-15 minutes. Serve the blend in unique dishes with the eggs coasting on the top.

Nutrition:

Calorie: 116

Protein: 6.97 g

Fat: 5.22 g

Carbohydrates: 13.14 g

Exquisite Turmeric Pancakes with Lemon Yogurt Sauce

Preparation time: 45 minutes
Cooking time: 15 minutes
Servings: 8 hotcakes

Ingredients:

For The Yogurt Sauce

1 cup plain Greek yogurt

1 garlic clove, minced

1 to 2 tablespoons lemon juice (from 1 lemon), to taste

¼ teaspoon ground turmeric

10 crisp mint leaves, minced

2 teaspoons lemon pizzazz (from 1 lemon)

For The Pancakes

2 teaspoons ground turmeric

1½ teaspoons ground cumin

1 teaspoon salt

1 teaspoon ground coriander

½ teaspoon garlic powder

½ teaspoon naturally ground dark pepper

1 head broccoli, cut into florets

3 enormous eggs, gently beaten

2 tablespoons plain unsweetened almond milk

1 cup almond flour

4 teaspoons coconut oil

Directions:

Make the yogurt sauce. Join the yogurt, garlic, lemon juice, turmeric, mint and pizzazz in a bowl. Taste and enjoy with more lemon juice, if possible. Keep in a safe spot or freeze until prepared to serve.

Make the flapjacks. In a little bowl, join the turmeric, cumin, salt, coriander, garlic and pepper.

Spot the broccoli in a nourishment processor, and heartbeat until the florets are separated into little pieces. Move the broccoli to an enormous bowl and include the eggs, almond milk, and almond flour. Mix in the flavor blend and consolidate well.

Heat 1 teaspoon of the coconut oil in a nonstick dish over medium-low heat. Empty ¼ cup player into the skillet. Cook the hotcake until little air pockets start to show up superficially and the base is brilliant darker, 2 to 3 minutes. Flip over and cook the hotcake for 2 to 3 minutes more. To keep warm, move the cooked hotcakes to a stove safe dish and spot in a 200°F oven.

Keep making the staying 3 hotcakes, utilizing the rest of the oil and player.

Nutrition:

Calories: 262

Protein: 11.68 g

Fat: 19.28 g

Carbohydrates: 12.06 g

Sirt Chili Con Carne

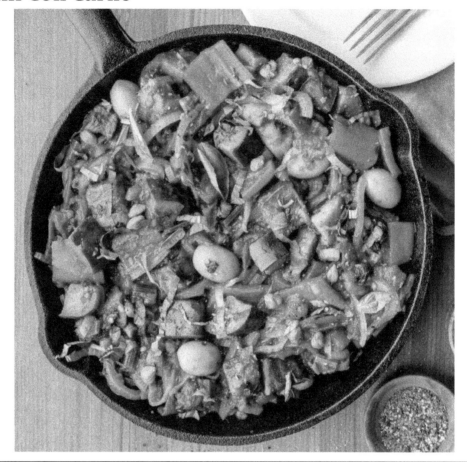

Preparation time: 1 hour 20 minutes
Cooking time: 1 hour 3 minutes
Servings: 4

Ingredients:

1 red onion, finely cleaved

3 garlic cloves, finely cleaved

2 10,000 foot chilies, finely hacked

1 tablespoon additional virgin olive oil

1 tablespoon ground cumin

1 tablespoon ground turmeric

400g lean minced hamburger (5 percent fat)

150ml red wine

1 red pepper, cored, seeds evacuated and cut into reduced down pieces

2 x 400g tins cleaved tomatoes

1 tablespoon tomato purée

1 tablespoon cocoa powder

150g tinned kidney beans

300ml hamburger stock

5g coriander, cleaved

5g parsley, cleaved

160g buckwheat

Directions:

In a meal, fry the onion, garlic and bean stew in the oil over a medium heat for 2-3 minutes, at that point include the flavors and cook for a moment.

Include the minced hamburger and dark colored over a high heat. Include the red wine and permit it to rise to decrease it considerably.

Include the red pepper, tomatoes, tomato purée, cocoa, kidney beans and stock and leave to stew for 60 minutes.

You may need to add a little water to accomplish a thick, clingy consistency. Just before serving, mix in the hacked herbs.

In the interim, cook the buckwheat as indicated by the bundle guidelines and present with the stew.

Nutrition:

Calories: 346 kcal

Protein: 14.11 g

Fat: 11.37 g

Carbohydrates: 49.25 g

Salmon and Spinach Quiche

Preparation time: 55 minutes
Cooking time: 45 minutes
Servings: 2

Ingredients:

600g frozen leaf spinach

1 clove of garlic

1 onion

150g frozen salmon fillets

200g smoked salmon

1 small Bunch of dill

1 untreated lemon

50 g butter

200 g sour cream

3 eggs

Salt, pepper, nutmeg

1 pack of puff pastry

Directions:

Let the spinach thaw and squeeze well.

Peel the garlic and onion and cut into fine cubes.

Cut the salmon fillet into cubes 1-1.5 cm thick.

Cut the smoked salmon into strips.

Wash the dill, pat dry and chop.

Wash the lemon with hot water, dry, rub the zest finely with a kitchen grater and squeeze the lemon.

Heat the butter in a pan. Sweat the garlic and onion cubes in it for approx. 2-3 minutes.

Add spinach and sweat briefly.

Add sour cream, lemon juice and zest, eggs and dill and mix well.

Season with salt, pepper and nutmeg.

Preheat the oven to 200 degrees top / bottom heat (180 degrees convection).

Grease a spring form pan and roll out the puff pastry in it and pull up on edge. Prick the dough with a fork (so that it doesn't rise too much).

Pour in the spinach and egg mixture and smooth out.

Spread salmon cubes and smoked salmon strips on top.

The quiche in the oven (grid, middle inset) about 30-40 min. Yellow gold bake.

Nutrition:

Calories: 903

Protein: 65.28 g

Fat: 59.79 g

Carbohydrates: 30.79 g

Choc Chip Granola

Preparation time: 55 minutes
Cooking time: 20 minutes
Servings: 2

Ingredients:

200g large oat flakes

Roughly 50 g pecan nuts chopped

3 tablespoons of light olive oil

20g butter

1 tablespoon of dark brown sugar

2 tablespoon rice syrup

60 g of good quality (70%)

Dark chocolate shavings

Directions:

Oven preheats to 160 ° C (140 ° C fan / Gas 3). Line a large baking tray with a sheet of silicone or parchment for baking.

In a large bowl, combine the oats and pecans. Heat the olive oil, butter, brown sugar, and rice malt syrup gently in a small non-stick pan until the butter has melted, and the sugar and syrup dissolve. Do not let boil. Pour the syrup over the oats and stir thoroughly until fully covered with the oats.

Spread the granola over the baking tray and spread right into the corners. Leave the mixture clumps with spacing, instead of even spreading. Bake for 20 minutes in the oven until golden brown is just tinged at the edges. Remove from the oven, and leave completely to cool on the tray.

When cold, split with your fingers any larger lumps on the tray and then mix them in the chocolate chips. Put the granola in an airtight tub or jar, or pour it. The granola is to last for at least 2 weeks.

Nutrition:

Calories: 914

Protein: 40.19 g

Fat: 63.05 g

Carbohydrates: 88.74 g

Aromatic Chicken Breast, Kale, Red Onion, and Salsa

Preparation time: 55 minutes
Cooking time: 30 minutes
Servings: 2

Ingredients:

120g skinless, boneless chicken breast

2 teaspoons ground turmeric

¼ lemon

1 tablespoon extra-virgin olive oil

50g kale, chopped

20g red onion, sliced

1 teaspoon fresh ginger, chopped

50g buckwheat

Directions:

To prepare the salsa, remove the tomato eye and finely chop. Add the chili, parsley, capers, lemon juice and mix.

Preheat the oven to 220ºC. Pour 1 teaspoon of the turmeric, the lemon juice and a little oil on the chicken breast and marinate. Allow to stay for 5–10 minutes.

Place an ovenproof frying pan on the heat and cook the marinated chicken for a minute on each side to achieve a pale golden color. Then transfer the pan containing the chicken to the oven and allow to stay for 8–10 minutes or until it is done. Remove from the oven and cover with foil, set aside for 5 minutes before serving.

Put the kale in a steamer and cook for 5 minutes. Pour a little oil in a frying pan and fry the red onions and the ginger to become soft but not colored. Add the cooked kale and continue to fry for another minute.

Cook the buckwheat following the packet's instructions using the remaining turmeric. Serve alongside the chicken, salsa, and vegetables.

Nutrition:

Calories: 149

Protein: 15.85 g

Fat: 5.09 g

Carbohydrates: 10.53 g

Braised Leek With Pine Nuts

Preparation time: 45 minutes
Cooking time: 15 minutes
Servings: 2

Ingredients:

20g Ghee

2 teaspoon Olive oil

2 pieces Leek

150 ml Vegetable broth

Fresh parsley

1 tablespoon fresh oregano

1 tablespoon Pine nuts (roasted)

Directions:

Cut the leek into thin rings and finely chop the herbs. Roast the pine nuts in a dry pan over medium heat.

Melt the ghee together with the olive oil in a large pan.

Cook the leek until golden brown for 5 minutes, stirring constantly.

Add the vegetable broth and cook for another 10 minutes until the leek is tender.

Stir in the herbs and sprinkle the pine nuts on the dish just before serving.

Nutrition:

Calories: 95

Protein: 1.35 g

Fat: 4.84 g

Carbohydrates: 12.61 g

Sweet and Sour Pan with Cashew Nuts

Preparation time: 30 minutes
Cooking time: 0 minutes
Servings: 2

Ingredients:

2 tablespoon Coconut oil

2 pieces Red onion

2 pieces yellow bell pepper

250 g White cabbage

150 g Pak choi

50 g Mung bean sprouts

4 pieces Pineapple slices

50 g Cashew nuts

For the sweet and sour sauce:

60 ml Apple cider vinegar

4 tablespoon Coconut blossom sugar

11/2 tablespoon Tomato paste

1 teaspoon Coconut-Amines

2 teaspoon Arrowroot powder

75 ml Water

Directions:

Roughly cut the vegetables.

Mix the arrow root with five tablespoons of cold water into a paste.

Then put all the other ingredients for the sauce in a saucepan and add the arrowroot paste for binding.

Melt the coconut oil in a pan and fry the onion.

Add the bell pepper, cabbage, pak choi and bean sprouts and stir-fry until the vegetables become a little softer.

Add the pineapple and cashew nuts and stir a few more times.

Pour a little sauce over the wok dish and serve.

Nutrition:

Calories: 573

Protein: 15.25 g

Fat: 27.81 g

Carbohydrates: 77.91 g

Vegetarian Paleo Ratatouille

Preparation time: 1 hour 10 minutes
Cooking time: 55 minutes
Servings: 2

Ingredients:

200 g Tomato cubes (can)

1 / 2 pieces Onion

2 cloves Garlic

1 / 4 teaspoon dried oregano

1 / 4 TL Chili flakes

2 tablespoon Olive oil

1 piece Eggplant

1 piece Zucchini

1 piece hot peppers

1 teaspoon dried thyme

Directions:

Preheat the oven to 180 ° C and lightly grease a round or oval shape.

Finely chop the onion and garlic.

Mix the tomato cubes with garlic, onion, oregano and chili flakes, season with salt and pepper and put on the bottom of the baking dish.

Use a mandolin, a cheese slicer or a sharp knife to cut the eggplant, zucchini and hot pepper into very thin slices.

Put the vegetables in a bowl (make circles, start at the edge and work inside).

Drizzle the remaining olive oil on the vegetables and sprinkle with thyme, salt and pepper.

Cover the baking dish with a piece of parchment paper and bake in the oven for 45 to 55 minutes.

Nutrition:

Calories: 273

Protein: 5.66 g

Fat: 14.49 g

Carbohydrates: 35.81 g

Frittata with Spring Onions and Asparagus:

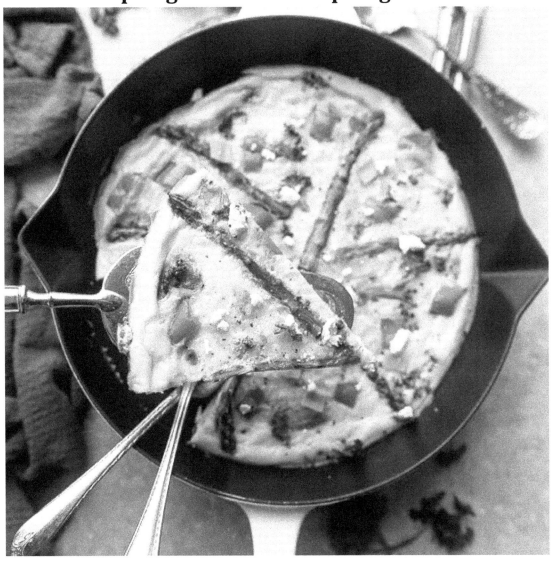

Preparation time: 15 minutes	
Cooking time: 10 minutes	
Servings: 2	

Ingredients:

5 pieces Egg

80 ml Almond milk

2 tablespoon Coconut oil

1 clove Garlic

100 g Asparagus tips

4 pieces Spring onions

1 teaspoon Tarragon

1 pinch Chili flakes

Directions:

Preheat the oven to 220 ° C.

Squeeze the garlic and finely chop the spring onions.

Whisk the eggs with the almond milk and season with salt and pepper.

Melt 1 tablespoon of coconut oil in a medium-sized cast iron pan and briefly fry the onion and garlic with the asparagus.

Remove the vegetables from the pan and melt the remaining coconut oil in the pan.

Pour in the egg mixture and half of the entire vegetable.

Place the pan in the oven for 15 minutes until the egg has solidified.

Then take the pan out of the oven and pour the rest of the egg with the vegetables into the pan.

Place the pan in the oven again for 15 minutes until the egg is nice and loose.

Sprinkle the tarragon and chili flakes on the dish before serving.

Nutrition:

Calories: 464 kcal

Protein: 24.23 g

Fat: 37.84 g

Carbohydrates: 7.33 g

Apple Pastry

Preparation time: 15 minutes
Cooking time: 30 minutes
Servings: 1

Ingredients:

Three cups all-purpose flour

Dash of salt

Two teaspoons margarine

One plain low-fat yogurt

One small apple

Dash each ground nutmeg and ground cinnamon

Two teaspoons reduced-calorie apricot spread (16 calories per 2 teaspoons)

Directions:

In a small mixing bowl, combine flour and salt; with a pastry blender, or two knives used scissors-fashion, cut in margarine until the mixture resembles a coarse meal. Add yogurt and mix thoroughly. Form dough into a ball; wrap in plastic wrap and refrigerate for at least 1 hour (maybe kept in the refrigerator for up to 3 days).

Between 2 sheets of a wax paper roll dough, forming a 4/2-inch circle about 1/2. Inch thick. Carefully remove wax paper and place dough on foil or small cookie sheet—Preheat oven to 350°F.

Core, pare, and thinly slice apple; arrange slices decoratively over the dough and sprinkle with nutmeg and cinnamon. Bake until crust is golden, 20 to 30 minutes.

During the last few minutes, that pastry is baking, in a small metal measuring cup or other small flameproof container heat apricot spread; as soon as the pie is done, brush with a warm space.

Nutrition:

238 calories;

4 g protein;

8 g fat;

38 g carbohydrate;

228 mg sodium;

1 mg cholesterol.

Baked Maple Apple

Preparation time: 10 minutes
Cooking time: 30 minutes
Servings: 2

Ingredients:

Two small apples

Two teaspoons reduced-calorie apricot

Spread

One teaspoon reduced-calorie maple-flavored syrup

Directions:

Remove the core from each apple to 1/2 inch from the bottom. Remove a thin strip of peel from around the center of each apple (this helps keep skin from bursting). Fill each apple with one teaspoon apricot spread and 1/2 teaspoon maple syrup. Place each apple upright in individual baking dish; cover dishes with foil and bake at 400°F until apples are tender, 25 to 30 minutes.

Nutrition:

75 calories; 0.2 g protein; 1 g fat;

19 g carbohydrate; 0.3 mg sodium;

Apple-Raisin Cake

Preparation time: 20 minutes
Cooking time: 50 minutes
Servings: 12

Ingredients: One teaspoon baking soda

1/2 cups applesauce (no sugar added)

Two small Golden Delicious apples, cored, pared, and shredded

1 cup less 2 s raisins

2/4 cups self-rising flour

1 teaspoon ground cinnamon

1/2 teaspoon ground cloves 1/3 cup plus 2 teaspoons unsalted margarine

1/4 cup granulated sugar

Directions:

Spray an 8 x 8 x 2-inch baking pan with nonstick cooking spray and set aside. Into a medium bowl sift together flour, cinnamon, and cloves; set aside.Preheat oven to 350°F. In a medium mixing bowl, using an electric mixer, cream margarine, add sugar and stir to combine. Stir baking soda into applesauce, then add to margarine mixture and stir to combine; add sifted ingredients and, using an electric mixer on medium speed, beat until thoroughly combined. Fold in apples and raisins; pour batter into the sprayed pan and bake for 45 to 50 minutes (until cake is browned and a cake tester or toothpick, inserted in center, comes out dry). Remove cake from pan and cool on wire rack.

Nutrition: 151 calories; 2 g protein;

4 g fat; 28 g carbohydrate; 96 mg sodium;

Cinnamon-Apricot Bananas

Preparation time: 45 minutes
Cooking time: 0 minutes
Servings: 2

Ingredients:

4 graham crackers 2x2-inch 1 medium banana, peeled and cut in squares), made into crumbs half lengthwise

2 teaspoons shredded coconut

1/4 teaspoon ground cinnamon

1 plus 1 teaspoon reduced-calorie apricot spread (16 calories per 2 teaspoons)

Directions:

In small skillet combine crumbs, coconut, and cinnamon and toast lightly, being careful not to burn; transfer to a sheet of wax paper or a paper plate and set aside.

In the same skillet heat apricot spread until melted; remove from heat. Roll each banana half in a spread, then quickly roll in crumb mixture, pressing crumbs so that they adhere to the banana; place coated halves on a plate, cover lightly, and refrigerate until chilled.

Variation: Coconut-Strawberry Bananas —Omit cinnamon and substitute reduced-calorie strawberry spread (16 calories per 2 teaspoons) for the apricot spread.

Nutrition:

130 calories; 2g protein;

2g fat; 29g carbohydrate;

95mg sodium;

Meringue Crepes with Blueberry Custard Filling

Preparation time: 10 minutes
Cooking time: 20 minutes
Servings: 4

Ingredients:

2 cups blueberries (reserve 8 berries for garnish)

1 cup evaporated skimmed milk

2 large eggs, separated

1 plus 1 teaspoon granulated sugar, divided

2 teaspoons each cornstarch

Lemon juice

Directions:

In 1-quart saucepan, combine milk, egg yolks, and one sugar; cook over low heat, continually stirring, until slightly thickened and bubbles form around sides of the mixture. In a cup or small bowl dissolve cornstarch in lemon juice; gradually stir into milk mixture and cook, constantly stirring, until thick. Remove from heat and fold in blueberries; let cool.

Spoon Vs. of custard onto the center of each crepe and fold sides over filling to enclose; arrange crepes, seam-side down, in an 8 x 8 x 2-inch baking pan. In a small bowl, using an electric mixer on high speed, beat egg whites until soft peaks form; add remaining teaspoon sugar, and continue beating until stiff peaks form.

Fill the pastry bag with egg whites and pipe an equal amount over each crepe (if pastry bag is not available, spoon egg whites over crepes); top each with a reserved blueberry and broil until meringue is lightly browned, 10 to 15 seconds. Serve immediately.

Nutrition:

300 calories;

16g protein;

6g fat;

45g carbohydrate;

180mg sodium;

278mg cholesterol

Chilled Cherry Soup

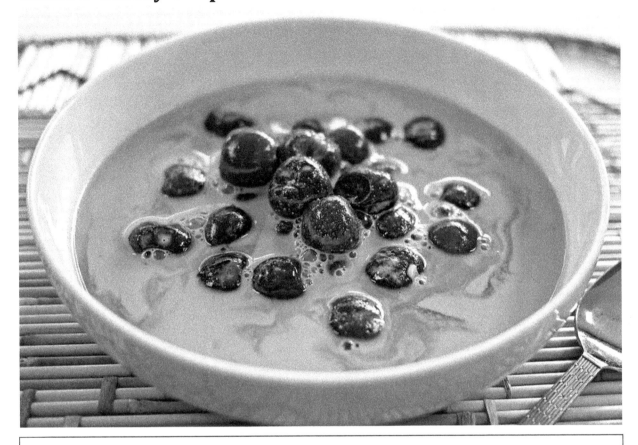

Preparation time: 5 minutes
Cooking time: 5 minutes
Servings: 2

Ingredients:

20 large frozen pitted cherries (no sugar added)

1/2 cup water

1/2 teaspoons granulated sugar

2-inch cinnamon stick

1 strip lemon peel

2 s rose wine

1 teaspoon cornstarch

1/4 cup plain low-fat yogurt

Directions:

In a small saucepan, combine cherries, water, sugar, cinnamon stick, and lemon peel; bring to a boil. Reduce heat, cover, and let simmer for 20 minutes.

Remove and discard the cinnamon stick and lemon peel from a cherry mixture. In measuring cup or small bowl combine wine and cornstarch, stirring to dissolve cornstarch; add to cherry mixture and, constantly stirring, bring to a boil. Reduce heat and let simmer until the mixture thickens.

In a heatproof bowl, stir yogurt until smooth; add cherry mixture and stir to combine. Cover with plastic wrap and refrigerate until well chilled

Nutrition:

98 calories;

2 g protein;

1 g fat;

19 g carbohydrate;

21 mg sodium;

2 mg cholesterol

Iced Orange Punch

Preparation time: 20 minutes
Cooking time: 0 minutes
Servings: 8

Ingredients:

Ice Mold Club soda

1 lemon, sliced 1 lime, sliced

Punch

1 quart each chilled orange juice (no sugar added), club soda, and diet ginger ale)

Directions:

To Prepare Ice Mold: Pour enough club soda into a 10- or 12-cup ring mold to fill mold; add lemon and lime slices, arranging them in an alternating pattern. Cover the mold and carefully transfer to freezer; freeze until solid.

To Prepare Punch: In a large punch bowl, combine juice and sodas. Remove ice mold from ring mold and float ice mold in a punch.

Nutrition:

56 calories; 1g protein; 0.1 g fat;

14 g carbohydrate; 35 mg sodium;

Meatless Borscht

Preparation time: 15 minutes
Cooking time: 45 minutes
Servings: 2

Ingredients: 1 teaspoon margarine

1 cup shredded green cabbage

1/4 cup chopped onion

1/4 cup sliced carrot

1 cup coarsely shredded pared

2 s tomato paste beets 1 lemon juice

2 cups of water

1/2 teaspoon granulated sugar

2 packets instant beef broth and 1 teaspoon pepper

Seasoning mix 1/2 bay leaf

1/4 cup plain low-fat yogurt

Directions: In 1 1/2-quart saucepan heat margarine until bubbly and hot; add onion and sauté until softened, 1 to 2 minutes. Add beets and toss to combine; add water, broth mix, and bay leaf and bring to a boil. Cover pan and cook over medium heat for 10 minutes; stir in remaining ingredients except for yogurt, cover, and let simmer until vegetables are tender about 25 minutes. Remove and discard bay leaf. Pour borscht into 2 soup bowls and top each portion with 2 s yogurt.

Nutrition: 120 calories; 5g protein; 3g fat;

21g carbohydrate; 982mg sodium;

2mg cholesterol

Sautéed Sweet 'N' Sour Beets

Preparation time: 10 minutes
Cooking time: 10 minutes
Servings: 2

Ingredients:

Serve hot or chilled.

2 teaspoons margarine

1 diced onion

1 cup drained canned small whole beets, cut into quarters

1 each lemon juice and water

1 teaspoon each salt and pepper

Dash granulated sugar substitute

Directions:

In small nonstick skillet heat margarine over medium-high heat until bubbly and hot; add onion and sauté until softened, 1 to 2 minutes. Reduce heat to low and add remaining ingredients; cover pan and cook, stirring once, for 5 minutes longer.

Nutrition:

70 calories;

1g protein;

4g fat;

9g carbohydrate;

385 mg sodium;

Orange Beets

Preparation time: 10 minutes
Cooking time: 10 minutes
Servings: 2

Ingredients:

1 /2 teaspoons lemon juice

1 teaspoon cornstarch Dash salt

1 teaspoon orange marmalade

1 cup peeled and sliced cooked beets

2 teaspoons margarine

1 teaspoon firmly packed brown

Sugar 1/4 cup orange juice (no sugar added)

Directions:

In a 1-quart saucepan (not aluminum or cast-iron), combine beets, margarine, and sugar; cook over low heat, continually stirring until margarine and sugar are melted.

In 1-cup measure or small bowl combine juices, cornstarch, and salt, stirring to dissolve cornstarch; pour over beet mixture and, constantly stirring, bring to a boil. Continue cooking and stirring

Until the mixture thickens.

Reduce heat, add marmalade, and stir until combined. Remove from heat and let cool slightly; cover and refrigerate for at least 1 hour. Reheat before serving.

Nutrition:

99 calories; 1g protein; 4g fat;

16g carbohydrate; 146mg sodium;

Cabbage 'N' Potato Soup

Preparation time: 10 minutes
Cooking time: 40 minutes
Servings: 4

Ingredients:

This soup freezes well; for easy portion control, freeze in pre-measured servings.

2 teaspoons vegetable oil

4 cups shredded green cabbage

1 cup sliced onions

1 garlic clove, minced

3 cups of water

6 ounces peeled potato, sliced

1 cup each sliced carrot and tomato puree

4 packets instant beef broth and seasoning mix

1 each bay leaf and whole clove

Directions:

In 2-quart saucepan heat oil, add cabbage, onions, and garlic and sauté over medium heat, frequently stirring, until cabbage is soft, about 10 minutes. Reduce heat to low and add remaining ingredients; cook until vegetables are tender, about 30 minutes. Remove and discard bay leaf and clove before serving.

Nutrition:

119 calories; 4 g protein; 3 g fat;

22 g carbohydrate; 900 mg sodium,

Eggplant Pesto

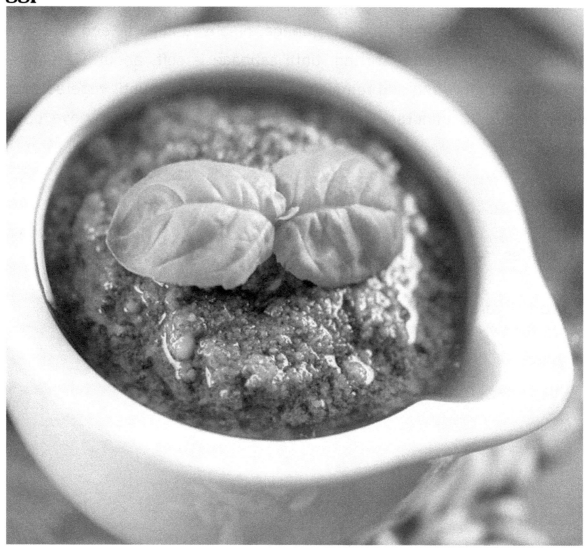

Preparation time: 15 minutes
Cooking time: 30 minutes
Servings: 2

Ingredients:

1 medium eggplant (about 1 pound), cut crosswise into thick rounds

Dash salt

Fresh basil and grated Parmesan cheese

1 olive oil

1 small garlic clove, mashed

Dash freshly ground pepper

Directions:

On 10 X 15-inch nonstick baking sheet arrange eggplant slices in a single layer; sprinkle with salt and bake at 425°F. Until easily pierced with a fork, about 30 minutes.

In a small bowl, combine remaining ingredients; spread an equal amount of mixture over each eggplant slice. Transfer slices to I1/2-quart casserole, return to oven, and bake until heated, about 10 minutes longer.

Nutrition:

144 calories;

5g protein;

9g fat;

14g carbohydrate;

163mg sodium;

4mg cholesterol

Chapter 2 Desserts Recipes

Snowflakes

Preparation time: 15 minutes
Cooking time: 10 minutes
Servings: 1

Ingredients:

Won ton wrappers

Oil to frying

Powdered sugar

Directions:

Cut won ton wrappers just like you'd a snowflake

Heat oil. When hot, add wonton, fry for approximately 30 seconds then flip over.

Drain on a paper towel and dust with powdered sugar.

Nutrition:

Calories: 96

Net carbs: 24.1g

Fat: 0.6g

Fiber: 5.3g

Protein: 2.8g

Home-Made Marshmallow Fluff

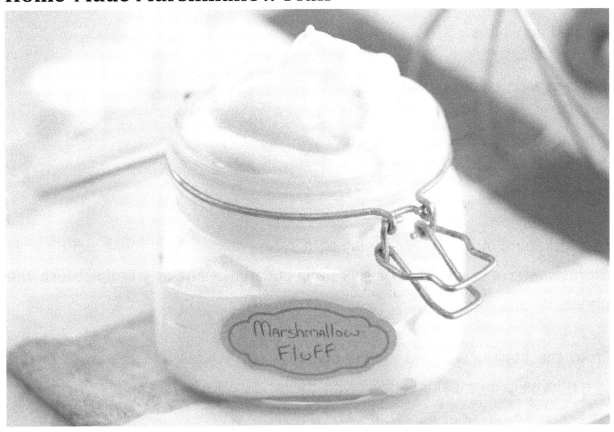

Preparation time: 15 minutes
Cooking time: 20 minutes
Servings: 4

Ingredients:

3/4 cup sugar

1/2 cup light corn syrup

1/4 cup water

⅛ Teaspoon salt

3 little egg whites

1/4 teaspoon cream of tartar

1 teaspoon 1/2 teaspoon vanilla extract

Directions:

In a little pan, mix together sugar, corn syrup, salt and water. Attach a candy thermometer into the side of this pan, but make sure it will not touch the underside of the pan.

From the bowl of a stand mixer, combine egg whites and cream of tartar. Begin to whip on medium speed with the whisk attachment.

Meanwhile, turn a burner on top and place the pan with the sugar mix onto heat. Pout mix into a boil and heat to 240 degrees, stirring periodically.

The aim is to have the egg whites whipped to soft peaks and also the sugar heated to 240 degrees at near the same moment. Simply stop stirring the egg whites once they hit soft peaks.

Once the sugar has already reached 240 amounts, turn heat low allowing it to reduce. Insert a little quantity of the popular sugar mix and let it mix. Insert still another little sum of the sugar mix. Add mix slowly and that means you never scramble the egg whites.

After all of the sugar was added into the egg whites, then decrease the speed of the mixer and also keep mixing concoction for around 7- 9 minutes until the fluff remains glossy and stiff. At roughly the 5-minute mark, then add the vanilla extract.

Use fluff immediately or store in an airtight container in the fridge for around two weeks.

Nutrition:

Calories: 23

Net carbs: 5.8g

Protein: 0.1g

Guilt Totally Free Banana Ice-Cream

Preparation time: 15 minutes
Cooking time: 0 minutes
Servings: 3

Ingredients:

3 quite ripe banana - peeled and chopped

A couple of chocolate chips

Two skim milk

Directions:

Throw all ingredients into a food processor and blend until creamy.

Eat: freeze and appreciate afterward.

Nutrition:

Calories: 387

Net carbs: 47.3g

Fat: 19.5g

Fiber: 1g

Protein: 6.3g

Perfect Little PB Snack Balls

Preparation time: 15 minutes
Cooking time: 0 minutes
Servings: 1

Ingredients:

1/2 cup chunky peanut butter

3 flax seeds

3 wheat germ

1 honey or agave

1/4 cup powdered sugar

Directions:

Blend dry ingredients and adding from the honey and peanut butter.

Mix well and roll into chunks and then conclude by rolling into wheat germ.

Nutrition:

Calories: 95

Net carbs: 6.6g

Fat: 5.6g

Fiber: 1.2g

Protein: 5.7g

Dark Chocolate Pretzel Cookies

Preparation time: 15 minutes
Cooking time: 20 minutes
Servings: 4

Ingredients:

1 cup yogurt

1/2 teaspoon baking soda

1/4 teaspoon salt

1/4 teaspoon cinnamon

4 butter (softened/0

1/3 cup brown sugar

1 egg

1/2 teaspoon vanilla

1/2 cup dark chocolate chips

1/2 cup pretzels, chopped

Directions:

Preheat oven to 350 degrees.

In a medium bowl whisk together the sugar, butter, vanilla and egg.

In another bowl, stir together the flour, baking soda, and salt.

Stir the bread mixture in, using all the wet components, along with the chocolate chips and pretzels until just blended.

Drop large spoonful of dough on an unlined baking sheet.

Bake for 15-17 minutes, or until the bottoms are somewhat all crispy.

Allow cooling on a wire rack.

Nutrition:

Calories: 300

Net carbs: 44.3g

Fat: 11.2g

Fiber: 1.3g

Protein: 3.8g

Marshmallow Popcorn Balls

Preparation time: 5 minutes
Cooking time: 20 minutes
Servings: 6

Ingredients: 2 bag of microwave popcorn

1 12.6 ounces. Tote M&M's

3 cups honey roasted peanuts

1 pkg. 16 ounce. Massive marshmallows

1 cup butter, cubed

Directions:

In a bowl, blend the popcorn, peanuts and M&M's. In a big pot, combine marshmallows and butter. Cook using medium-low heat. Insert popcorn mix, blend thoroughly Spray muffin tins with non-stick cooking spray.

When cool enough to handle, spray hands together with non-stick cooking spray and then shape into chunks and put into the muffin tin to shape. Add Popsicle stick into each chunk and then let cool.

Wrap each serving in vinyl when chilled.

Nutrition:

Calories: 36 Net carbs: 7.4g Fat: 0.2g

Fiber: 0.3g Protein: 0.9g

Home-Made Ice-Cream Drumsticks

Preparation time: 15 minutes
Cooking time: 0 minutes
Servings: 4

Ingredients:

Vanilla ice cream

Two Lindt hazelnut chunks

Magical shell - out chocolate

Sugar levels

Nuts (I mixed crushed peppers and unsalted peanuts)

Parchment paper

Directions:

Soften ice cream and mixing topping - I had two sliced Lindt hazelnut balls.

Fill underside of Magic shell with sugar and nuts and top with ice-cream.

Wrap parchment paper round cone and then fill cone over about 1.5 inches across the cap of the cone (the paper can help to carry its shape).

Sprinkle with magical nuts and shells.

Freeze for about 20 minutes, before the ice cream is eaten.

Nutrition:

Calories: 267

Net carbs: 32.4g Fat: 14.2g Fiber: 0.9g

Protein: 4.6g

Ultimate Chocolate Chip Cookie N' Oreo Fudge Brownie Bar

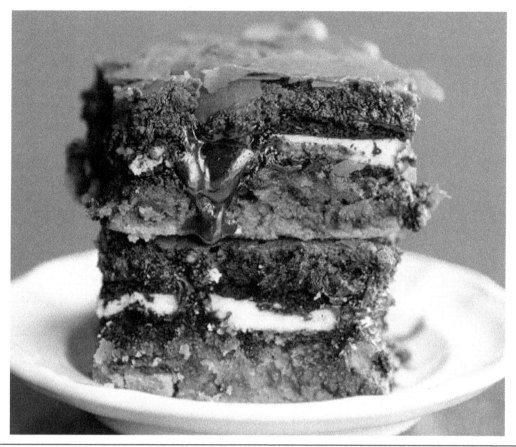

Preparation time: 20 minutes
Cooking time: 70 minutes
Servings: 4

Ingredients:

1 cup (2 sticks) butter, softened

1 cup granulated sugar

3/4 cup light brown sugar

2 large egg

1 pure vanilla extract

2 ½ cups all-purpose flour

1 teaspoon baking soda

1 teaspoon lemon

2 cups (12 Oz) milk chocolate chips

1 package double stuffed Oreo

1 family-size (9×1 3) brownie mixture

1/4 cup hot fudge topping

Directions:

Preheat oven to 350 degrees F.

Cream the butter and sugars in a large bowl using an electric mixer at medium speed for 35 minutes.

Add the vanilla and eggs and mix well to combine thoroughly. In another bowl, whisk together the flour, baking soda and salt, and slowly incorporate in the mixer everything is combined.

Stir in chocolate chips.

Spread the cookie dough at the bottom of a 9×1-3 baking dish that is wrapped with wax paper and then coated with cooking spray.

Shirt with a coating of Oreos. Mix together brownie mix, adding an optional 1/4 cup of hot fudge directly into the mixture.

Stir the brownie batter within the cookie-dough and Oreos.

Cover with foil and bake at 350 degrees F for 30 minutes.

Remove foil and continue baking for another 15 25 minutes.

Let cool before cutting on brownies. They may be gooey at the while warm but will also set up perfectly once chilled.

Nutrition:

Calories: 181

Net carbs: 30g

Fat: 5.4g

Fiber: 1.1g

Protein: 3g

Crunchy Chocolate Chip Coconut Macadamia Nut Cookies

Preparation time: 15 minutes
Cooking time: 5 minutes
Servings: 5

Ingredients:

1 cup yogurt 1 cup yogurt

1/2 teaspoon baking soda

1/2 teaspoon salt

1 of butter, softened

1 cup firmly packed brown sugar

1/2 cup sugar

1 large egg

1/2 cup semi-sweet chocolate chips

1/2 cup sweetened flaked coconut

1/2 cup coarsely chopped dry-roasted macadamia nuts

1/2 cup raisins

Directions:

Preheat the oven to 325ºf.

In a little bowl, whisk together the flour, oats and baking soda and salt; then place aside.

In your mixer bowl, mix together the butter/sugar/egg mix.

Mix in the flour/oats mix until just combined and stir into the chocolate chips, raisins, nuts, and coconut.

Place outsized bits on a parchment-lined cookie sheet.

Bake for 1-3 minutes, before biscuits are only barely golden brown.

Remove from the oven and then leave the cookie sheets to cool at least 10 minutes.

Nutrition:

Calories: 317 Net carbs: 20.5g

Fat: 9.9g Fiber: 2.3g Protein: 35.2g

Peach and Blueberry Pie

Preparation time: 20 minutes
Cooking time: 60 minutes
Servings: 4

Ingredients:

1 box of noodle dough

Filling:

5 peaches, peeled and chopped (I used roasted peaches)

3 cups strawberries

3/4 cup sugar

1/4 cup bread

Juice of 1/2 lemon

1 egg yolk, beaten

Directions:

Preheat oven to 400 degrees.

Place dough to a 9-inch pie plate

In a big bowl, combine tomatoes, sugar, bread, and lemon juice, then toss to combine. Pour into the pie plate, mounding at the center.

Simply take some of bread and then cut into bits, then put a pie shirt and put the dough in addition to pressing on edges.

Brush crust with egg wash then sprinkles with sugar. Set onto a parchment paper-lined baking sheet. Bake at 400 for about 20 minutes, until crust is browned at borders.

Turn oven down to 350, bake for another 40 minutes. Remove and let sit at least 30minutes.

Have with vanilla ice-cream.

Nutrition:

Calories: 360 Net carbs: 49.2g

Fat: 17.4g Protein: 3.9g

Pear, Cranberry And Chocolate Crisp

| Preparation time: 15 minutes |
| Cooking time: 40 minutes |
| Servings: 4 |

Ingredients:

Crumble topping:

1/2 cup flour

1/2 cup brown sugar

1 teaspoon cinnamon

⅛ Teaspoon salt

3/4 cup yogurt

1/4 cup sliced peppers

1/3 cup butter, melted

1 teaspoon vanilla

Filling:

1 brown sugar

3 teaspoon, cut into balls

1/4 cup dried cranberries

1 teaspoon lemon juice

Two handfuls of milk chocolate chips

Directions:

Preheat oven to 375.

Spray a casserole dish with a butter spray.

Put all of the topping ingredients - flour, sugar, cinnamon, salt, nuts, legumes and dried

Butter a bowl and then mix. Set aside.

In a large bowl combine the sugar, lemon juice, pears, and cranberries.

Once the fully blended move to the prepared baking dish.

Spread the topping evenly over the fruit.

Bake for about half an hour.

Disperse chocolate chips out at the top.

Cook for another 10 minutes.

Have with ice cream.

Nutrition:

Calories: 418 Net carbs: 107.7g

Fat: 0.4g Fiber: 2.8g Protein: 0.5g

Apricot Oatmeal Cookies

Preparation time: 10 minutes
Cooking time: 40 minutes
Servings: 7

Ingredients:

1/2 cup (1 stick) butter, softened

2/3 cup light brown sugar packed 1 egg

3/4 cup all-purpose flour

1/2 teaspoon baking soda

1/2 teaspoon vanilla extract

1/2 teaspoon cinnamon 1/4 teaspoon salt

1 teaspoon 1/2 cups chopped oats

3/4 cup yolks 1/4 cup sliced apricots

1/3 cup slivered almonds

Directions:

Preheat oven to 350°. In a big bowl combine with the butter, sugar, and egg until smooth. In another bowl whisk the flour, baking soda, cinnamon, and salt together. Stir the dry ingredients to the butter-sugar bowl. Now stir in the oats, raisins, apricots, and almonds.

I heard on the web that in this time, it's much better to cool with the dough (therefore, your biscuits are thicker)

Nutrition:

Calories: 196 Net carbs: 30g

Fat: 8.1g Fiber: 0.5g Protein: 3g

Raw Vegan Reese's Cups

Preparation time: 10 minutes
Cooking time: 35 minutes
Servings: 4

Ingredients:

"Peanut" butter filling

½ cup sunflower seeds butter

½ cup almond butter

1 raw honey

2 melted coconut oil

Super foods chocolate part:

½ cup cacao powder

2 raw honey

1/3 cup of coconut oil (melted)

Directions:

Mix the "peanut" butter filling ingredients.

Put a spoonful of the mixture into each muffin cup.

Refrigerate.

Mix super foods chocolate ingredients.

Put a spoonful of the super foods chocolate mixture over the "peanut" butter mixture. Freeze!

Nutrition:

Calories: 549 Net carbs: 54g Fat: 31.7g

Fiber: 2.1g Protein: 11.8g

Raw Vegan Coffee Cashew Cream Cake

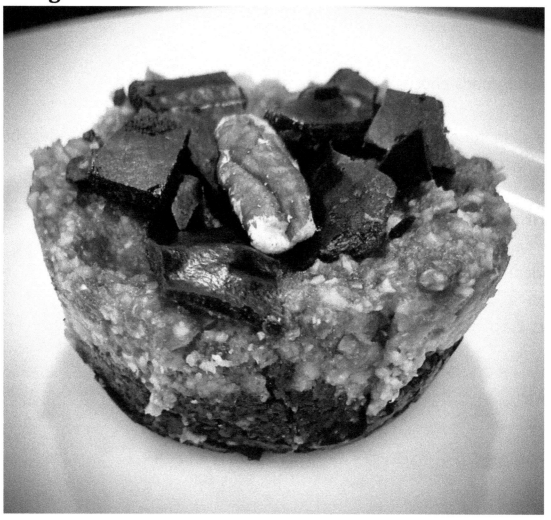

Preparation time: 10 minutes
Cooking time: 35 minutes
Servings: 4

Ingredients:

Coffee cashew cream

2 cups raw cashews

1 teaspoon of ground vanilla bean

3 melted coconut oil

¼ cup raw honey

1/3 cup very strong coffee or triple espresso shot

Directions:

Blend all ingredients for the cream, pour it onto the crust and refrigerate.

Garnish with coffee beans.

Nutrition:

Calories: 94

Net carbs: 4.4g

Fat: 7.9g

Fiber: 0.3g

Protein: 2.8g

Raw Vegan Chocolate Cashew Truffles

Preparation time: 10 minutes
Cooking time: 35 minutes
Servings: 4

Ingredients:

1 cup ground cashews

1 teaspoon of ground vanilla bean

½ cup of coconut oil

¼ cup raw honey

2 flax meal

2 hemp hearts

2 cacao powder

Directions:

Mix all ingredients and make truffles. Sprinkle coconut flakes on top.

Nutrition:

Calories: 87

Net carbs: 6g

Fat: 6.5g

Fiber: 0.5g

Protein: 2.3g

Raw Vegan Double Almond Raw Chocolate Tart

Preparation time: 10 minutes
Cooking time: 35 minutes
Servings: 4

Ingredients:

1½ cups of raw almonds

¼ cup of coconut oil, melted

1 raw honey or royal jelly

8 ounces dark chocolate, chopped

1 cup of coconut milk

½ cup unsweetened shredded coconut

Directions:

Crust:

Ground almonds and add melted coconut oil, raw honey and combine.

Using a spatula, spread this mixture into the tart or pie pan.

Filling:

Put the chopped chocolate in a bowl, heat coconut milk and pour over chocolate and whisk together.

Pour filling into tart shell.

Refrigerate.

Toast almond slivers chips and sprinkle over tart.

Nutrition:

Calories: 101 Net carbs: 3.4g Fat: 9.4g

Fiber: 0.6g Protein: 2.4g

Raw Vegan Bounty Bars

Preparation time: 10 minutes
Cooking time: 35 minutes
Servings: 4

Ingredients:

"Peanut" butter filling

2 cups desiccated coconut

3 coconut oil - melted

1 cup of coconut cream - full fat

4 of raw honey

1 teaspoon ground vanilla bean

Pinch of sea salt

Super foods chocolate part:

½ cup cacao powder 2 raw honey

1/3 cup of coconut oil (melted)

Directions:

Mix coconut oil, coconut cream, and honey, vanilla and salt.

Pour over desiccated coconut and mix well.

Mold coconut mixture into balls, small bars similar to bounty and freeze.

Or pour the whole mixture into a tray, freeze and cut into small bars.

Make super foods chocolate mixture, warm it up and dip frozen coconut into the chocolate and put on a tray and freeze again.

Nutrition:

Calories: 70 Net carbs: 6.7g Fat: 4.3g

Fiber: 0.2g Protein: 1g

Raw Vegan Tartlets with Coconut Cream

Preparation time: 10 minutes
Cooking time: 35 minutes
Servings: 4

Ingredients:

Pudding:

1 avocado

2 coconut oil

2 raw honey

2 cacao powder

1 teaspoon ground vanilla bean

Pinch of salt

¼ cup almond milk, as needed

Directions:

Blend all the ingredients in the food processor until smooth and thick.

Spread evenly into tartlet crusts.

Optionally, put some goji berries on top of the pudding layer.

Make the coconut cream, spread it on top of the pudding layer, and put back in the fridge overnight.

Serve with one blueberry on top of each tartlet.

Nutrition:

Calories: 200 Net carbs: 25.2g Fat: 4.3g

Fiber: 4.6g Protein: 12.8g

Raw Vegan "Peanut" Butter Truffles

Preparation time: 10 minutes
Cooking time: 30 minutes
Servings: 4

Ingredients:

5 sunflower seed butter

1 coconut oil

1 raw honey

1 teaspoon ground vanilla bean

¾ cup almond flour

1 flaxseed meal

Pinch of salt

1 cacao butter

Hemp hearts (optional)

¼ cup super-foods chocolate

Directions:

Mix until all ingredients are incorporated.

Roll the dough into 1-inch balls, place them on parchment paper and refrigerate for half an hour (yield about 14 truffles).

Dip each truffle in the melted super foods chocolate, one at the time.

Place them back on the pan with parchment paper or coat them in cocoa powder or coconut flakes.

Nutrition:

Calories: 94 Net carbs: 3.1g Fat: 8g

Fiber: 1g Protein: 4g

Raw Vegan Chocolate Pie

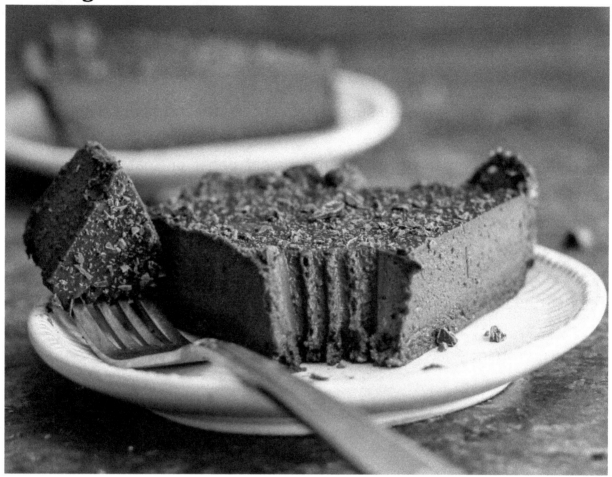

Preparation time: 10 minutes
Cooking time: 25 minutes
Servings: 4

Ingredients: Crust:

2 cups almonds, soaked overnight and drained

1 cup pitted dates, soaked overnight and drained

1 cup chopped dried apricots

1½ teaspoon ground vanilla bean

2 teaspoon chia seeds 1 banana

Filling:

4 raw cacao powder 3 raw honey

2 ripe avocados 2 organic coconut oil

2 almond milk (if needed, check for consistency first)

Directions:

Add almonds and banana to a food processor or blender.

Mix until it forms a thick ball.

Add the vanilla, dates, and apricot chunks to the blender.

Mix well and optionally add a couple of drops of water at a time to make the mixture stick together.

Spread in a 10-inch dis.

Mix filling ingredients in a blender and add almond milk if necessary.

Add filling to the crust and refrigerate.

Nutrition:

Calories: 380

Net carbs: 50.2g

Fat: 18.4g

Fiber: 2.2g

Protein: 7.2g

Raw Vegan Chocolate Walnut Truffles

Preparation time: 10 minutes
Cooking time: 35 minutes
Servings: 4

Ingredients:

1 cup ground walnuts

1 teaspoon cinnamon

½ cup of coconut oil

¼ cup raw honey

2 chia seeds

2 cacao powder

Directions:

Mix all ingredients and make truffles.

Coat with cinnamon, coconut flakes or chopped almonds.

Nutrition:

Calories: 120

Fat: 13.6g

Raw Vegan Carrot Cake

Preparation time: 10 minutes
Cooking time: 35 minutes
Servings: 4

Ingredients: Crust:

4 carrots, chopped 1½ cups oats

½ cup dried coconut 2 cups dates

1 teaspoon cinnamon ½ teaspoon nutmeg

1½ cups cashews 2 coconut oil

Juice from 1 lemon 2 raw honey

1 teaspoon ground vanilla bean

Water, as needed

Directions:

Add all crust ingredients to the blender.

Mix well and optionally add a couple of drops of water at a time to make the mixture stick together.

Press in a small pan.

Take it out and put on a plate and freeze.

Mix frosting ingredients in a blender and add water if necessary.

Add frosting to the crust and refrigerate.

Nutrition:

Calories: 241 Net carbs: 28.4g

Fat: 13.4g Fiber: 0.8g Protein: 2.4g

Frozen Raw Blackberry Cake

Preparation time: 10 minutes
Cooking time: 45 minutes
Servings: 4

Ingredients: Crust:

3/4 cup shredded coconut

15 dried dates soaked in hot water and drained

1/3 cup pumpkin seeds 1/4 cup of coconut oil

Middle filling Coconut whipped cream

Top filling:

1 pound of frozen blackberries

3-4 raw honey 1/4 cup of coconut cream

2 egg whites

Directions:

Grease the cake tin with coconut oil and mix all base ingredients in the blender until you get a sticky ball. Press the base mixture in a cake tin. Freeze. Make Coconut Whipped Cream. Process berries and add honey, coconut cream and egg whites. Pour middle filling - Coconut Whipped Cream in the tin and spread evenly. Freeze. Pour top filling - berries mixture-in the tin, spread, decorate with blueberries and almonds and return to freezer.

Nutrition:

Calories: 472 Net carbs: 15.8g Fat: 18g

Fiber: 16.8g Protein: 33.3g

Raw Vegan Chocolate Hazelnuts Truffles

Preparation time: 10 minutes
Cooking time: 30 minutes
Servings: 4

Ingredients:

1 cup ground almonds

1 teaspoon ground vanilla bean

½ cup of coconut oil

½ cup mashed pitted dates

12 whole hazelnuts

2 cacao powder

Directions:

Mix all ingredients and make truffles with one whole hazelnut in the middle.

Nutrition:

Calories: 370

Net carbs: 66.9g

Fat: 11.8g

Fiber: 2.6g

Protein: 4.2g

Raw Vegan Chocolate Cream Fruity Cake

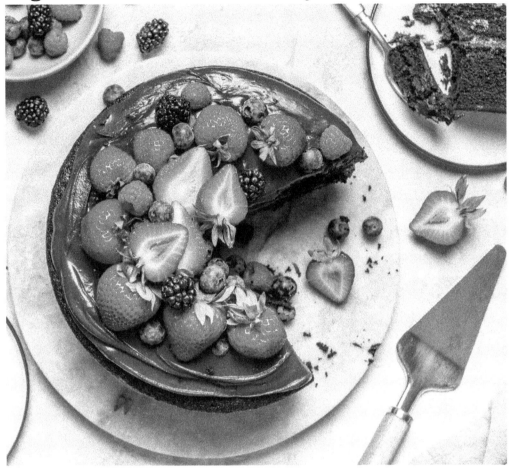

Preparation time: 10 minutes
Cooking time: 45 minutes
Servings: 4

Ingredients:

Chocolate cream: 1 avocado

2 raw honey 2 coconut oil

2 cacao powder

1 teaspoon ground vanilla bean

Pinch of sea salt

¼ cup of coconut milk

1 coconut flakes

Fruits:

1 chopped banana

1 cup pitted cherries

Directions:

Prepare the crust and press it at the bottom of the pan.

Blend all chocolate cream ingredients, fold in the fruits and pour in the crust.

Whip the top layer, spread and sprinkle with cacao powder.

Refrigerate.

Nutrition:

Calories: 106 Net carbs: 0.4g Fat: 5g

Fiber: 0.1g Protein: 14g

Jerusalem Artichoke Gratin

Preparation time: 10 minutes
Cooking time: 45 minutes
Servings: 3

Ingredients:

600g Jerusalem artichoke

250ml of milk

2 grated cheese

1 crème fraiche

1 butter

Curry, paprika powder, nutmeg, salt, pepper

Directions:

Wash and peel the Jerusalem artichoke tubers and slice them into approx. 3 mm thick slices. Bring them to a boil with the milk in a saucepan. Then stir in the spices and crème fraiche.

Grease a baking dish with butter and add the Jerusalem artichoke and milk mixture. Bake on the middle shelf in the oven for about half an hour at 160 °

C. Sprinkle with grated cheese and bake five minutes before the end of the baking time. Gorgeous!

Nutrition:

Calories: 133

Net carbs: 9.9g

Fat: 8.1g

Fiber: 1.1g

Protein: 4.7g

Baked Quinces With A Cream Crown

Preparation time: 20 minutes
Cooking time: 90 minutes
Servings: 1

Ingredients:

1-2 quinces

70-80 g whipped cream

1 teaspoon sugar

1 teaspoon vanilla sugar

Directions:

After you have freed the quince from its fluff, you wrap it loosely in aluminum foil and put it in the oven at 200 ° C for 60 to 90 minutes, the thicker the fruit, the longer the baking time.

Spend the wait waiting to whip the cream stiff and sweeten it.

When the quinces have softened, halve them, remove the core with a small spoon and then pour the sweet whipped cream into this trough.

Nutrition:

Calories: 52

Net carbs: 14g

Fiber: 1.7g

Protein: 0.3g

Apple And Pear Jam With Tarragon

Preparation time: 15 minutes
Cooking time: 0 minutes
Servings: 3

Ingredients:

500g juicy pears

500g sour apples

1 large lemon

2 sprigs of tarragon

500g jam sugar 2: 1

Directions:

Peel and quarter apples and pears, remove the core and dice or grate very, very finely.

Squeeze the lemon and add to the fruit with the gelling sugar.

Let the juice soak overnight!

Wash and dry the tarragon. Finely chop the leaves and add to the fruit mix.

Nutrition:

Calories: 242

Net carbs: 15g

Fat: 20.5g

Fiber: 3.2g

Protein: 2g

Apple Jam With Honey And Cinnamon

Preparation time: 10 minutes
Cooking time: 15 minutes
Servings: 2

Ingredients:

300g apples

6 lemon juice

2 sticks of cinnamon

50 g liquid honey,

500g jam sugar 2: 1

Directions:

Peel and quarter the apples and remove the core.

Weigh 1 kg of pulp. Dice this finely and drizzle with lemon juice.

Mix the pulp, gelling sugar and cinnamon sticks well in a large saucepan.

After cooking remove the cinnamon sticks and stir in the honey.

Nutrition:

Calories: 193 Net carbs: 38g Fat: 4.5g

Fiber: 1.8g Protein: 1.8g

Plum Chutney

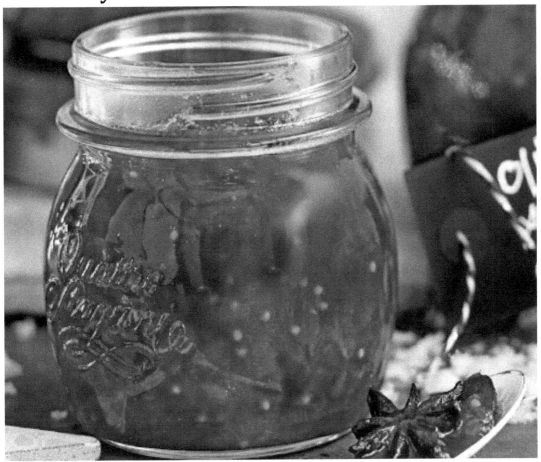

Preparation time: 5 minutes
Cooking time: 50 minutes
Servings: 4

Ingredients:

500 g pitted prunes

50 g ginger

350 g onions

2 s vegetable oil

250g brown sugar

300ml balsamic vinegar

Salt, pepper

Directions:

Quarter the washed and pitted plums. Finely dice the ginger and onions and braise in 2 s of oil. Add the plums and steam briefly.

Add the brown sugar and let it melt while stirring. Then pour balsamic vinegar over it and let it boil for about 40 minutes on a low flame.

Season with salt and pepper and pour into boiled glasses.

Nutrition:

Calories: 125

Net carbs: 19.6g

Fat: 4.9g

Fiber: 0.8g

Protein: 1.7g

Chocolate Chip Gelato

Preparation time: 30 minutes
Cooking time: 0 minutes
Servings: 4

Ingredients:

2 cups dairy-free milk

¾ cup pure maple syrup

1 pure vanilla extract

⅓ Semi-sweet vegan chocolate chips, finely chopped or flaked

Directions:

Beat dairy-free milk, maple syrup, and vanilla together in a large bowl until well combined.

Pour the mixture carefully into the container of an automatic ice cream maker and process it according to the manufacturer's instructions.

During the last 10 or 15 minutes, add the chopped chocolate and continue processing until the desired texture is achieved. Enjoy the gelato immediately, or let it harden further in the freezer for an hour or more.

Nutrition:

Calories: 94

Net carbs: 14.9g

Fat: 3.4g

Fiber: 0.5g

Protein: 0.8g

Peanut Butter And Jelly Ice Cream

Preparation time: 40 minutes
Cooking time: 0 minutes
Servings: 6

Ingredients:

2 cups dairy-free milk, simple, sugar-free

⅔ Cup maple syrup

3 s creamy natural peanut butter

½ teaspoon ground ginger

2 teaspoons pure vanilla extract

6 spoons canned fruits

Directions:

Beat the milk without milk, maple syrup, peanut butter, and vanilla in a large bowl until well combined. Pour the mixture carefully into the container of an automatic ice cream maker and process it according to the manufacturer's instructions.

Add canned fruits for the last 10 minutes, and let them combine with the ice cream until the desired texture is achieved. Enjoy the ice cream immediately, or let it harden further in the freezer for an hour or more.

Nutrition: Calories: 189 Net carbs: 33.8g

Fat: 4.1g Fiber: 0.7g Protein: 5.6g

Watermelon Gazpacho In A Jar

Preparation time: 20 minutes
Cooking time: 0 minutes
Servings: 8

Ingredients:

1kg of ripe, aromatic tomatoes

Half a red pepper +

Half a small chili pepper

3 ground cucumbers

1 onion

1 clove of garlic (optional)

2 cups cubed watermelon

Juice of 1 lemon

A handful of leaves basil

A handful of mint leaves

1 - 2 s olive oil

Salt, pepper

Directions:

Tomato peel slightly cut in several places, then transfer the tomatoes to a deep pot and pour boiling water, let stand for a few minutes. Drain the water and peel the tomatoes from the skin, but this is not a necessary stage if the skin does not bother you. Peeled tomatoes in half and put in a blender cup or larger bowl. Add chopped onion, garlic, diced peppers, cucumbers, chili peppers, and lemon juice. Also, add basil and mint leaves. All mix well in a blender or using a hand blender, finally adding olive oil.

Then add chopped pieces of watermelon and mix only for a moment, so that the remaining watermelon particles can be felt. Season with salt and pepper to taste.

Serve well chilled with diced paprika, lemon juice, stale bread, and a large dose of fresh, chopped basil.

Nutrition:

Calories: 46

Net carbs: 4.3g

Fat: 0.2g

Fiber: 0.5g

Protein: 7g

Conclusion

Thank you for making it to the end, it would be nice to get some feedback from you regarding these quick recipes to stay in shape without having to give up the pleasure of eating your favorite dishes.

Remember that this diet does not only aim at slimming but also at physical well-being, look for the best way to activate your metabolism, and remember that this diet regime is a real anti-aging regime, in fact these diets take advantage of a series of foods that allow the activation of a hormone called sirtuin that can have a wide range of health benefits, as well as muscle building and appetite suppression. There is strong observational evidence for the beneficial effects of consuming foods and beverages, rich in sirtuin activators, in reducing the risks of chronic disease.The beauty of these snak and dessert recipes will allow you to have fun and lose weight at the same time, which will allow you to lose weight in a calm and relaxed manner without having to reduce yourself to stressful and frustrating situations. Have fun and enjoy your diet.

CPSIA information can be obtained
at www.ICGtesting.com
Printed in the USA
BVHW091615300321
603711BV00007B/1255